Made in the USA
Middletown, DE
31 May 2020

96426155R10057